WEIGHT LOSS WITH THE NORDIC DIET

SAGA FINBERG

Dedicated to Shalga Breen
Thank you for being such a wealth of info,
support and encouragement.

Disclaimer

You may also enjoy:

HOROSCOPE 2015: Astrology and Numerology Horoscopes

The mystery/thrillers:

A Sealed Fate

Holly Leaves

Next of Sin

As well as (all in ebook and paperback):

Gluten-Free Mediterranean Diet for Beginners: 25 Delicious Recipes from the Healthiest Region in the World – Sophie Miller

Healthy Slow Cooker Recipes: 50 Easy Winter Warming Recipes for Breakfast, Lunch, Dinner, and Dessert! – Sophie Miller

Gluten-Free Bread: Delicious Easy Homemade Bread – Sopjie Miller

Delicious, Nutritious Recipes for the Time and Cash Strapped Paleo Diet: Get Started, Get Motivated, Feel Great. – Lisa Lazuli_BESTSELLER

99 ACE Places to Promote Your Book - Lisa Lazuli

Pressure Cooking Reinvented – Lisa Lazuli – BEST SELLER

SUGAR FREE DESSERTS WITH PAZAZ – Lisa Lazuli - NEW

Weight Loss with the Nordic Diet – Saga Finberg - NEW

Be Wine Savvy – Joelle Nevin - NEW

Contents

CONVERSION TABLES (Metric and Imperial)

METRIC	IMPERIAL
5 ml	1 teaspoon – tsp
15 ml	1 Tablespoon – Tbs
60 ml	¼ cup
80 ml	1/3 cup
120ml	½ cup
160 ml	2/3 cup
180 ml	¾ cup
240 ml	1 cup
480 ml	2 cups
568ml	1 pint
250 grams	9 oz
500 g	1 lb 2 oz
1 kg	2 lb 3 oz
160 C	320 F
180 C	360 F
200 C	400 F

Courgettes = zucchini = baby marrow
Aubergine = eggplant = brinjal
Tin Foil = Aluminium Foil

What is The Nordic Diet?

Chow down like a Viking ... and lose weight ... and be fully satisfied. How can this be? It's called the Nordic Diet, and it's among the latest trends in dieting and healthy eating that's good for you AND satisfying too! From the delicious salmon delicacy and distinctly North country dish called Gramavlax, to Icelandic Lamb Kabobs and Beetroot Tartar with chicken liver and apples, you'll enjoy every bite down the Viking road. (Medianet author, June)

First, what is the Nordic, sometimes called New Nordic, Diet? It's based on local and seasonal Scandinavian cuisine that includes free-range meats, wild fish and game, vegetables that are cold-climate hardy, wild berries, and whole grains. These ingredients are chock full of healthful vitamins and are all very helpful in weight loss and a disease-free life. In many ways, the Nordic Diet is similar to the vaunted Mediterranean Diet, but includes food that is native to cold climates.

Even though this diet is intended to help prevent cardiovascular disease, it can also prevent obesity and Type-2 Diabetes as well as cancer.

There are 3 basic guidelines for the Nordic Diet:

1. Get more of your food from oceans and lakes. Shellfish and fish of all kinds, are high in protein and beneficial fats. Using more of these resources can help prevent cardiovascular disease, obesity, and Type II diabetes. Because these seafoods contain a large amount of protein, they can also prevent age-related loss of musculature in older adults.

   There are two types of fish – fatty and lean. Alternate between the two to get the most benefit out of fish and shellfish. The different types contain differing amounts of omega 3 fatty acids, vitamins, and minerals. Also, alternating can help prevent risks of illness related to mercury pollution.

2. More of the calories we eat should be obtained from plants than meat. High protein intake is beneficial and can help overweight, older, and sedentary people to prevent disease, but meat is not environmentally friendly, and that is an integral part of the diet. Meat takes much more water and plant input per calorie than vegetables, grains, and fruit. By eating more plants in place of meat, we will minimize our intake of saturated fat, one of the leading causes of cardiovascular disease. This will also increase our consumption of vitamins, minerals, fiber and healthy fats. Because plants are lower in calories, we can eat more of them to ensure fullness yet lower the calories that we consume.

3. An important aspect of the Nordic Diet, and one of its most noticeable, is that many foods are obtained from the wild. Foraged meat, berries, and mushrooms are very healthy because they contain much higher

portions of the antioxidant vitamins. Wild fowl and animals are almost always less fatty than their domestic counterparts, and contain less saturated fat especially. Instead, they are rich in a much higher proportion of Omega 3 fatty acids, which are much healthier.

Is the Nordic Diet a good choice?

There have only been a few studies of the Nordic Diet, and two of them are presented here to show that the diet is effective and compares favorably to similar diets such as the Mediterranean Diet.

Journal of Internal Medicine Study (Hansen, 2012)

A study conducted in the Nordic countries of Denmark, Finland, Sweden, and Iceland, examined the health effects of the Nordic Diet on vital signs including blood fat profile, Type 2 Diabetes sensitivity, inflammation, and blood pressure. The study included 166 Scandinavians from these countries, all white, and all with metabolic syndrome (obesity, insulin resistance, Type 2 Diabetes, high Body Mass Index) and was published in the Journal of Internal Medicine.

Participants followed either a standard diet of red meat, potatoes, and white bread, or a Nordic diet consisting of poultry, fish, nuts, and local produce and vegetables. The Nordic diet was very similar to the cuisine of Rene Rezepi, featured below, of the restaurant Noma, a world famous purveyor of Scandinavian cuisine. The people that followed the Nordic avoided meat, other than fish, sugar, sausages, and pastries. They focus on local plants, wild animals, and fish such as lutefisk and pickled herring.

The Nordic Diet followed by the participants emphasized these principles:

- Fruits of any king, but including apples, pears, and plums
- Vegetables like legumes, root vegetable, and cabbage
- Barley, rye, and oats. Whole grains made up no less than 25 percent of the diet
- Berries, to include native berries such as black currants, bilberries, and strawberries
- Rapeseed (canola) oil for cooking
- Low-fat dairy
- Fish at least 3 times per week
- Low fat white or game meat such as poultry and wild game
- Drinks that do not contain sugar.

The group on the standard diet did not follow any of these principals. They used butter, far fewer fruits and vegetables, less fish, poultry, and game. In addition, there were no limits on flour, sugar and red meat. Both diets had a similar calorie count, but differed in the salt, fiber, and fat intake, according to researchers. Other than the stated differences, all participants were required to maintain the normal activity, whether or not that included smoking, drinking, and minimal activity. If the participants were previously active, they were to remain that way.

The results of the study determined that the Nordic Diet improves health in the following ways:

- Lowers cholesterol

   Participants in the study who followed the Nordic diet portion of the plan had much lower levels of the potentially harmful LDECILITER (low-density lipoprotein) cholesterol, and much higher levels of the potentially beneficial HDECILITER (high-density lipoprotein) cholesterol when compared to those who did not follow the Nordic portion of the diet.

- Compares favorably to the Mediterranean Diet

Like the better-known Mediterranean diet, the Nordic Diet involves healthy eating, to include lots of vegetables, fruits, lean proteins, and whole grains. Butter and fat oils are not allowed in large quantities, and olive oil or rapeseed (canola) oil are preferred instead.

- Prevents Cognitive Decline

Cognitive Decline and early death have been shown to be caused by sugar, red meat, and flour or refined grains. The Nordic Diet fits the "Harvard Healthy Plate" criteria for healthy eating which recommends lots of fish, canola oil, nuts, legumes, grains, vegetables, and fruits, and emphasizes avoiding additional sugar, dairy, and red meat. Research shows that the Nordic Diet can help prevent Cognitive Decline.

--

Meinert Larsen Study (Dr. Thomas Meinert Larsen, 2012)

In the Meinert Larsen Study, the key was to eat only food in season, so for instance, dinner in the spring might be baked cod with celery, while in the summer it might be pike grilled with summer cabbage.

Scientists at Copenhagen University sought inspiration for Nordic diet recipes from chefs at Noma, the local restaurant designated the best in the world, who have spent the last decade encouraging people to eat seasonal, local foods, and forage for their salads.

The study led by Dr Thomas Meinart Larsen, who works at the university's OPUS center, involved the following adults:

- 181 overweight adults who were asked to eat one of two different diets for six months.

- Altogether 68 people were assigned to an 'average Danish diet', comprised of the dishes currently most eaten in Denmark, including many imported foods.

- The remaining 113 people were put on the New Nordic Diet, with Meyer-designed recipes with ingredients made up of local and seasonal whole foods.

All of the participants were encouraged to eat until they were fully satisfied, paying some attention to portion size, but never counting calories.

Those randomized to the Nordic diet received a cookbook with 180 recipes with three menu plans for each season, while those randomized to the Danish diet received a cookbook with 99 recipes but no menu plans - since seasonal variation was not important. Dr Meinart Larsen said 'One innovative aspect of the study was that all ingredients were provided free of charge at a special shop.' The food taken away was registered on computer and if it did not conform to the assigned diet, the customer was asked to change their choices. The actual cost of the Nordic diet was around £4.75 a day, about a quarter more costly than the average diet.

Results showed those in the Nordic diet group improved their health.

- The participants lost around 4.7kg (10 pounds) on average compared with a loss of 1.5kg (three pounds) for the Danish diet group.
- The Nordic diet also produced greater cuts in systolic (-5.1 mm Hg) and diastolic blood pressure (-3.2 mmHg) than the Danish diet.

Dr Meinart Larsen, speaking at the European Society of Cardiology meeting in Barcelona, Spain, said the reduction were important to the individuals, and could make a big difference if it were repeated across the population, since even small long-term blood pressure reductions will reduce cardiovascular deaths.

The concept of a healthy, regional, sustainable, seasonal and highly palatable diet, he added, could in principle be applied anywhere in the world, not just Nordic countries.

Berries, fresh herbs, mushrooms, plants, and even seaweed are collected from the wild, and whole grains are used in conjunction with potatoes, cabbages, legumes and root vegetables. Greater consumption of fish, including turbot and wild salmon, decreases the amount of meat included in the diet, although fresh game such as deer and musk ox may be eaten. "Our view is that eating foods in accordance with the seasons makes us less dependent on transportation" he said.

"There's particular emphasis on foraged foods because they taste better, and usually contain greater amounts of vitamins and minerals than conventionally grown plants" he added. He said the impetus for developing the diet came from the difficulties in integrating the heart-healthy Mediterranean diet into the regular eating habits of the Danes, who have a distinctly different food history.

Greater use of fish, including wild salmon and turbot, reduces the amount of meat included in the diet, although fresh game such as deer and musk ox may be eaten. In fact, the Danes had one of the worst records for heart disease until deaths started plummeting a decade ago – a change attributed to a ban against added industrially produced transfat acids to processed foods in 2003. The Average Danish Diet comprised of food typically found on Danish supper tables and in Danish lunch packs, including meat balls, pizza and spaghetti with meat sauce. The ingredients are often dairy products, potatoes, bread, pasta, rice, meat and vegetables such as tomatoes and cucumber. Teaching children to cook local ingredients is included in the OPUS research project, and the goal is that the New Nordic Diet becomes the twenty-first century's response to the Mediterranean diet, as per Dr Meinart Larsen.

A bit of History – The story of Redzepi's (Hansen, 2012)

This story is included because it is a prime example of the Nordic Diet and how it has been exported to the larger world. This fun description of the use of ants exemplifies the manner in which the Nordic Diet obtains food from the wild. Also, Mr. Rezepi is a world-renowned champion of the Nordic Diet and lifestyle.

In August 2012, the Danish restaurant Noma, along with its head chef René Redzepi, went to London to share with the British his ideas on fine food and ants, for a fortnight. (Hansen, 2012)

During the Olympic Games, the world famous Danish restaurant Noma moved into the luxurious setting of Claridge's Hotel in London.

Ten days later, there were 3,500 reservations for a table, all booked within two hours. After that, Richard Vines, food critic for Bloomberg, wanted to know if this was adequate proof that the notions of what had, by that time, become identified as the "new Nordic kitchen", had been transferred to another country.

Noma's head chef and co-owner René Redzepi's reply to this question was that the philosophy and enthusiasm known, could now be adopted anywhere.

The method that René Redzepi brought with him to London is based on a constant search for new fields in gastronomy, and he is happy to take new and surprising ingredients into use. In London, he did not hesitate in treating his guests to live ants. They taste, according to the Danish chef, of lemongrass.

As a general rule, Redzepi only uses local ingredients – and preferably ingredients that he and the rest of the staff at Noma have gathered themselves. The focus is on sustainability, respect for nature and using original foods which Redzepi thinks are disappearing with the industrialization of our food culture.

"We try to make food with the ingredients we have around us. We work with local farmers, we gather local ingredients that Nature provides – and we exploit seasonal ingredients to the limit," says Redzepi, who insists that it is not about idealizing the past or returning to the Stone Age: "Naturally not. We use the most modern machinery – anything else would be silly."

René Redzepi has often been compared with the Danish film director Lars von Trier, who in the 1990s established the golden age of Danish film, based on a strict set of rules concerning the use of the handheld camera, and the non-use of artificial light and sound, scenography and costumes.

In the same way, a Nordic dogma for cooking has developed where the rules include the use of local ingredients, and dishes that must reflect the changing seasons while at the same time being based on modern knowledge concerning the connection between health and tastiness. The rules also include promoting the wellbeing and sustainability of animals in relation to our natural resources.

This approach put René Redzepi on the front page of Time Magazine earlier this year under the headline "Locavore Hero". The magazine used the term "Redzepi effect" to describe chefs who apply the dogma of geographical limitation in the ingredients they use.

"I don't want to be quoted here and there for saying that you have to do such and such. I don't want to judge other people, they can do as they please, because I do what I want. In reality there is nothing particularly sacred about my menu. I actually just recreated the meals I grew up with, as a child, in Macedonia. We lived largely on vegetables and livestock from the family farm, so when we were served chicken it was really a big thing.

Slaughtering was not something that happened every day, so it was very natural that vegetables represented the largest part of the meal," he says.

René Redzepi grew up in Denmark, but his father's family is originally from Macedonia, where René spent his summers until the war in the Balkans broke out in 1992. His family background and the summer holidays in Macedonia provide, according to the chef himself, a good part of the explanation for why he makes food the way he does.

"In Macedonia the whole family lived in the same house, where everything centered around the main meal of the day. The whole day was used to prepare the evening meal – people were farmers and if chicken was on the menu, we had to slaughter it first. If we wanted milk, we had to milk the cow," says Redzepi.

It is this authenticity and genuineness in food preparation that has brought success to René Redzepi and Noma. Nikolaj Stagis, whose book The Authentic Company includes interviews with Redzepi, agrees with this. Stagis has followed Redzepi's career since Noma opened in 2003.

The explanation offered by Nikolaj Stagis is that even though many thought that Noma's Nordic dogma would be a short-lived fashion, it has turned out to be a feasible concept because the people running the restaurant do not become complacent and rest on their laurels, but continue to refine and promote what they are really good at.

"An authentic company works with something original – something old-fashioned, historic or in another way a carrier of our heritage. But it also changes the historic features, it revolutionizes or innovates at the same time. It reflects on its own material and takes it forward," says Nikolaj Stagis with reference to Noma.

After the Olympic Games in London, René Redzepi and the rest of Noma's staff are back in Copenhagen. The London experience has been digested, and Redzepi can look back on ten intense days with lots of international star status, celebrities at the tables and autograph hounds.

"Here at home it is not like that at all. It's funny, but in London you can achieve an almost surreal star status if you are a successful chef. It was wild and slightly overwhelming, and I have perhaps been a bit shy. But I think you just have to be yourself and then enjoy the moment."

Weight Loss with the Nordic Diet

The studies cited above show that the Nordic Diet improves the levels of blood cholesterol in people facing cardiovascular risks, compared to the usual Danish diet or a diet typical to Western standards. Some studies have determined that the Nordic Diet reduces blood pressure and decreases insulin sensitivity.

Participants in studies who were on the diet for between 6 and 20 weeks benefitted from the improvements.

An interesting side effect of the studies showed that participants enjoyed significant weight loss, indicating that they were satisfied with the food, even though they weren't calorie restricted. This shows that eating the natural foods of the Nordic Diet can help people lose weight without even trying!

In addition, participants who ate the foods recommended in the Nordic Diet had a much lower risk of premature death over a period of 12 years.

Nordic Diet Food List

Oily Fish

Oily or fatty fish that are packed with Omega 3 fatty acids are key to this diet. They help brain development, control blood sugar, and protect against cardiovascular disease. These foods are especially good for physical development in children and are plentiful in the northern countries of Denmark, Finland, Sweden, and Norway. These vitamin and fatty acid rich foods include salmon, herring, and mackerel, and they should be a staple of the diet.

Canola Oil

Known as rapeseed oil in Nordic countries, canola oil is their main oil for cooking. It is used instead of olive oil, prevalent in the Mediterranean diet, because it is more available in the Nordic regions. Either canola or olive oil can be used in the Nordic Diet.

Both of these oils contain just 6 to 14 percent saturated fat, which is far lower than the saturated fat found in butter. If canola oil is used, it is also a very good source of vitamin C.

Berries

The Nordic countries grow many types of berries, and all are incorporated into the diet. Some of these may not be available in many countries, but most of them are. These berries include

- Blueberries
- Wild Strawberries
- Black and Red Currants
- Lingonberries
- Elderberries
- Cloudberries

Interestingly, people in Nordic countries add berries to fish and meat, or eat them plain or in deserts. Some of these deserts can be found in the recipes section. Berries are full of antioxidants to prevent diseases such as cardiovascular disease, strokes, and cancer, caused by free radicals.

Wild Meat

Venison is the term for the meat of wild animals such as deer, reindeer, and elk, which are hunted, and this type of meat is preferred in the Nordic Diet. This can make the diet expensive unless the family hunts their own meat, but poultry, organic substitutes, or other lean meat can be substituted and is much easier to find in Western groceries.

Whole Grains

Rather than the highly processed white bread commonly found in the Western diet, breads made of whole wheat, rye, and oats are recommended. Whole grains have been found to reduce the risk of cancer, obesity, Type II Diabetes, and cardiovascular disease.

Fruits and Vegetables

Fruits and vegetables are very important to the Nordic Diet and can be eaten whole, hot, cold, or as a side dish. With this diet, fruits are commonly incorporated into meat dishes, and starchy plants such as potatoes can be boiled. These foods are good sources of vitamins and minerals.

How to adopt the Nordic Diet

Any diet that is rich in fruits and vegetables, fish, lean meats, and whole grains is very healthful, especially when refined grains and flour, sugar, fatty red meat, and processed foods are avoided. The Nordic Diet, therefore, is this set of principles expressed in the cuisine of the Nordic region of the world.

These basic components can be incorporated in the American interpretation of the Nordic Diet by visiting local farmer's markets or becoming a member of a food co-op or Community Supported Agriculture farm. These places give Americans and other Westerners greater access to berries, plants, and wild game. And of course, ants are available anywhere.

Some of the basic principles:

- Buy local and organic
- Buy seasonal produce
- Avoid processed foods

- Make the bulk of your diet whole grains like rye, barley, oats, and whole wheat

- Eat lots of nuts, seeds, beans, and food from the wild like wild game and mushrooms

- Make fish a large part of your diet

- Reduce the red meat that is commercially produced

- Eat lean, grass-fed, cage-free, and free-range meat, eggs, and cheese whenever possible

Recipes

For other great recipes and more information about Nordic meals, see "The Principles of Good Flavor" by Claus Meyer of Noma Restaurant.

Appetizers and Quick Meals

Cabbage and Salmon salad

1 Cabbage finely shredded (I recommend a heart shaped cabbage, if you use a savoy make sure you shred finely)
1 Braeburn or Granny Smith apple cored, quartered then sliced.
½ English Cucumber, peeled and sliced
1 bunch dill
1 Celery stick finely sliced
Salmon (tinned or fresh)

Sauce:
2 Tbs chopped onion
1 cup canola oil
½ cup brown sugar
½ cup brown vinegar or cider vinegar
1 tsp mustard
1 tsp celery salt

Method
1. Whisk sauce ingredients together and leave for two hours so flavours blend.
2. Mix cabbage, apple, dill, cucumber and celery together in a salad bowl. Top with salmon and then drizzle dressing oil over.

Creamy Millet with Pickled Onions, Mushrooms, and Grated
Cheddar

Pickled onions
4-5 shallots
2 tsp cold-pressed canola oil
4 Tbs raw honey
4 Tbs wine vinegar
Finely chopped red pepper
Tarragon
salt and pepper

Millet
10 oz pearl millet or quinoa (I often mix the two using 5 oz each)
2 small onions
2 Tbs cold-pressed hemp oil
4-5 cups chicken or vegetable stock (or water)

Asparagus, Zucchini and Mushroom Mix
3 Shallots
14 oz. Mixed mushrooms ie button or dried chanterelles, porcini,
portobellos
14.1 oz fine asparagus (do not use thick stemmed asparagus
which needs to be steamed)
15 oz zucchini/ baby marrow julienne
1 Tbs hemp oil
½ tsp sage
2.1 oz firm cheese, like "Red Leicester", "Gloucester", "Cheddar"
or "Gruyere"
Whole meal bread

Method
1. Cut the shallots in half lengthways. Sauté onions gently in
canola oil, until golden. Add wine vinegar, tarragon, red pepper
and honey then simmer until the majority of the liquid has
evaporated (takes approx. 10 min). Season with salt and pepper.

2. Place millet (or millet quinoa mix) into a sieve and rinse off
well under running water.

Finely chop the onions and sauté in oil in frying pan, until the onions are soft and transparent. Add the millet mix, stir in well. Add the stock, and simmer for another 20 minutes until the mixture is creamy. Season with salt and ground black pepper.

3. Halve the larger mushrooms lengthwise and leave smaller ones whole. If you are using dried mushrooms, soak in boiling water for 30 mins to one hour before cooking. Cut asparagus sticks into 3-4 pieces, discarding ends. Fry the mushrooms, zucchini and asparagus in the hemp oil, season with salt, pepper and sage as soon as you start frying and cook over high heat for approx. 2 minutes stirring constantly.

4 Mix the pickled onions with the millet, top the millet with the fried mushroom mix in casserole dish, grate cheese on top and heat dish for 10-15 mins in a hot oven (180C). Serve with wholegrain bread.

Skagen Herring

20 salt herrings
2 cups diced onion
2 cups diced apples
2 cups canola or hemp oil
Pepper to taste
1 small tin tomato puree
Bay leaves
¼ cup brown sugar
2 tsp mustard

Method:
1. Soak herrings overnight in cold water. Clean and remove all bones. Cut into ½ inch squares.
2. Mix oil, sugar, vinegar and tomato puree. Then add apples, herring pieces and onion and mix. Finally add bay leaves and mustard.
3. This keeps for many days if refrigerated and can be brought out as a starter or snack. Remove herrings from liquid and herbs and serve with brown bread pieces or biscuits.

Skyla Tuna Salad

240 g/ 8.4 oz tinned tuna, drained
1/2 c finely chopped cooked cauliflower
1 cup canned green beans chopped
1 Tbs capers
1/2 tsp paprika
1/2 tsp garlic powder
2 Tbs mayonnaise
2 Cos lettuce leaves

Method
1. Mix first 4 ingredients and toss.
2. Add paprika and garlic powder to mayonnaise and mix.
3. Add mayonnaise to tuna mixture and serve on lettuce leaves.

Anjali Pilchard Mouse

500g / 1 lb tin pilchards (skinned, boned and mashed)
½ c boiling water
1 tsp prepared mustard
2 eggs separated
Salt and pepper
1 Tbs gelatine
1 tsp sugar
½ c dry white wine or vinegar
½ c mayonnaise

Method:
1. Soak gelatine in cold water. Then dissolve in ½ c boiling water.
2. Put beaten egg yolks, sugar, salt, mustard and wine into a double boiler and cook until mixture coats spoon (stirring all the while).
3. Cool mixture slightly.
4. Add dissolved gelatine and chill until about to set. Add fish and mayonnaise and mix.
5. Fold in stiffly beaten egg whites.
6. Turn into a wet mould and chill.

Brilliant for having with seeded biscuits, ryevita, on rice cakes or crackers.

Nichola's Fried Stuffed Herring

2lb / 800g Fresh Herrings
1 ½ tsp Salt
3 Tbs Butter
½ cup parsley
1 egg beaten
½ breadcrumbs
½ cup canola oil

Method
1. Clean fish, removing heads and tails. Rinse in cold water and drain. Split, bone and leave whole.
2. Spread out, skin side down and sprinkle with salt.
3. Cream butter with parsley and spread on half of the fish, top with remaining fish to form sandwiches.
4. Dip in beaten egg then coat with breadcrumbs.
5. Heat oil, sauté fish on both sides until golden brown.

Serve with mashed potatoes and a salad. Mix a spoonful of wholegrain mustard into your mashed potato as this goes brilliantly with the herrings.

Delicious serves with Riesling, Muscat or Sauvignon Blanc.

Chicken Liver Pate

250 g/ 8 oz chicken livers
2 medium onions
3 Tbs Canola Oil
2 hard-boiled eggs
4 tsp matzos meal or fine bread crumbs
Salt and pepper

Method:
1. Fry onions and liver in 3 Tbs oil until soft.
2. Cool then blend with one of the eggs.
3. Add matzos meal and oil from frying pan to liver.
4. Season, mix and add more oil if necessary. Blend again.
5. Put in shallow dish and cover with chopped egg.

Serve with seed bread, chutney and rocket leaves.

Herrings in Cream

5 salt herrings
1 large onion
1 cup vinegar
3 bay leaves
6 peppercorns
1/2 tsp mustard
2 tsp sugar
3 eggs
300ml/ 1/2 pint sour cream

Method:
1. Soak herrings overnight. Fillet and put in a flat dish.
2. Cover with sliced onion.
3. Boil vinegar, bay leaves, mustard sugar and peppercorns. Cool. Add three well beaten eggs and mix with vinegar. Strain and cool.
4. Add cream and pour over herrings.
5. Refrigerate for 24 hours then serve with sour dough bread.

Malmo Potato Salad

500g/ 1lb peeled potatoes halved
1 onion grated
2 hard-boiled eggs
1 Tbs mixed dried rosemary, parsley and sage
1 cup mayonnaise
½ tsp mustard
Squeeze lemon juice
5-8 herrings in brine
Salt and white pepper

Method:

1. Steam the potatoes and allow to cool.
2. Slice the eggs.
3. Mix the mayonnaise with the lemon, herbs and mustard.
4. Dice cool potatoes, place in a bowl and mix in sliced egg, onion and mayonnaise.
5. Rinse and chop herrings and arrange on top

Mackerel with Hazelnuts

1 cup red quinoa or millet or brown rice
¾ cup water
1 cup fresh peas
1 cup yoghurt
Juice from ½ lemon
¼ cup chopped parsley or dill
½ cup hazelnuts and cashew nuts mixed
½ cup cold pressed canola oil
4 smoked mackerels
Rocket leaves
Salt and pepper

Method
1. Wash rocket.
2. Rinse quinoa (or millet/rice) and place in boiling water and cook with a little salt until tender, which takes 15-20 mins.
3. Boil the peas for 5 minutes and then place into a blender and blend. Add yoghurt and dill, then blend again. Sprinkle with lemon juice, salt and pepper

4. Place hazelnuts and cashew nuts on a baking tray, sprinkle with canola oil so nuts are covered and roast for 10 mins. Allow the nuts to cool, season and then blend them with canola oil for about 10 seconds to make a paste.

5. Grill mackerel. .

6. Serve mackerel on a bed of rocket and quinoa, with the pea purée and hazelnut paste on the side.

Chicken Livers with Beetroot Salad

60g / 2 oz butter
1 large onion chopped
1 small clove crushed garlic
150 ml/ ¼ pint double cream
2 eggs lightly beaten
4 Tbs chicken stock
500g/ 1 lb chicken livers
Salt and freshly ground black pepper
1 level tsp cornflower
4 Tbs dry sherry
60g/ 2 oz melted butter

Method
1. Melt butter, add onion, garlic and stock, bring to boil and simmer gently for 10 mins or until onion is soft.
2. Trim livers and add to onion and stock with salt and ground black pepper.
3. Simmer for 10 mins over low heat.
4. Pass liver and liquid thru a blender.
5. Mix cream, eggs , cornflower and sherry then stir into liver blend.
6. Place into a well-greased corning dish/pyrex and cover with foil.
7. Place this dish into a shallow baking dish with water in it so the water come 1" up the sides.
8. Back for 2-2 ½ hours at 160C. Remove from oven and allow to cool. Top with melted butter when cool. Chill for 24 hours.

Beetroot Salad

1 green apple
½ cup chopped celery
2 Tbs chopped walnuts

¾ cup mayoniase
2 beetroots, cooked and diced
Shredded romaine lettuce
Horseradish

Method
Combine apple, celery and walnuts with mayonnaise. Pour over
beetroot and toss well adding extra mayo if needed. Arrange on
lettuce.

Serve pate and beetroot salad with generous amount of
wholegrain brown bread and horseradish.

Potato and Leek Soup

Soup

500 gram/ 1lb potatoes, peeled and diced
2 leeks, chopped
2 onions, chopped
Bunch of fresh chives chopped
3 cloves garlic, crushed
2 Tbs cold-pressed hemp or canola oil
3 pints chicken or vegetable stock
¼ tsp celery salt
salt and ground black pepper
1-2 Tbs thick cream

Method:

1. Place all the vegetables into a large saucepan and fry gently for 10 mins over low heat, do not allow vegetables to burn. Season with celery salt, salt and black pepper. Add the stock (or just use boiling water).
2. Boil for one hour. Separate into portions allow to cool and then blend. Reheat the portions you need for that meal and stir in a Tbs per serving of cream before serving.

Beautiful with Rye Bread.

Potato Soup with Nettles

Soup

500g / 1lb peeled diced potatoes
1 large onion
1 leek chopped
7 oz /200 g watercress
1 Tbs canola oil
1 litre or 2 pints vegetable stock
100 gram nettles (the shoots found in early srping are the best, but buds from older plants can be used)
Chervil
Salt and pepper
250 ml or 1 cup Coconut milk -

Method

1. Fry the onion gently in a large saucepan in the canola oil until clear, which should take about 15 min then add the watercress and cook gently for another 10 -15 mins.
2. Introduce the potatoes, chervil, leek and water into another pot and simmer gently for 30 mins. Then rinse nettles and stir in, before adjusting the flavor with salt and pepper and cooking another 5 mins.
3. Add the onions and watercress to the potato mixture. Cook for another 10 mins.
4. Cool slightly and blend. Stir in ½ cup cream or coconut cream to create a beautifully smooth texture.

Halland Beetroot Soup

4 Large beetroots
Salt, pepper and sugar
600ml/ 1 pint chicken stock
1 400g/ 14 oz carton plain yoghurt
1 stick celery chopped finely
1 onion chopped finely
Garlic granules
2 Tbs thick cream if desired.

Method:
1. Cook the beetroots in water with some salt, pepper and sugar. A pressure cooker works well if you have one. Otherwise cover with water, place lid on and boil until tender.
2. When cooked, cool and then place in blender with a small amount of the stock. You can lightly fry the finely chopped onion and add to the beetroot before blending to give more body.
3. Add stock, celery and yoghurt. Blend again.
4. Add salt, pepper and garlic granules.
5. Heat well. Only stir in cream when you have removed soup from heat, just before serving.

Coquina Soup

500 g/ 1 lb Coquina butternut squash or sweet potatoes or a mixture of both
2 leeks, chopped
2 carrots chopped
2 onions, chopped
2 garlic cloves, crushed
400g/ 14 oz Tin butter beans
2 pints chicken or vegetable stock although water is fine
100g or 3.5 oz pearly barley
½ tsp turmeric
Bunch of coriander/ Cilantro chopped
1 cup coconut cream
½ cup sesame seeds

Method

1. Place chopped onion, leeks, carrot and squash into a saucepan. Add stock/water and bring to boil. Season with salt and ground black pepper, add garlic, turmeric and coriander.
2. Boil for 1 hour. Add barley and boil for another 15-20 minutes, until barley is clear. Add the tin of butter beans and then boil for another 5 minutes.
3. Remove from heat, cool slightly and then blend.
4. Place sesame seed on a baking tray and toast lightly.
5. Stir coconut cream into soup and serve immediately with toasted sesame seed sprinkled on top.

Fish Chowder

500g/ 1lb Maris Piper or Charlotte potatoes, peeled and diced
2-3 leeks, chopped
2 Tbs hemp oil
1 large onion, chopped
2 cloves garlic, crushed
2 pints chicken or fish stock
1 bouquet garni
300 g/ 10.5 oz thick smoked hake fillets, warmed
Salt and ground black pepper
Stale French loaf
Parsley and garlic salt

Method
1. Place potatoes, onions and leeks into a large saucepan and sauté them gently for a few minutes at low heat. Add garlic and season with salt and pepper.
2. Pour in the stock and bouquet garni and let simmer for 35-40 minutes, until the potatoes and leeks are tender.
3. Then remove from heat, cool slightly and blend the leek and potato soup.
4. Pour blended soup back into the pot. Break the smoked fish into large pieces, add it to the soup and bring to a boil.

Cut French bread into cubes. Melt some butter. Add finely chopped parsley and garlic salt to the butter and stir well. Fry the French bread cubes in the butter mix. It works better when the bread is slightly stale.

Bergen Barley Broth

500g/ 1lb neck of mutton
2 pints cold water
Fresh Rosemary and Thyme
Salt and Pepper
2 Tbs chopped parsley
2 Tbs pearl barley
1 Carrot chopped
1 Turnip chopped
1 parsnip chopped
1 onion chopped.

Method
1. Put mutton, salt, pepper, thyme and rosemary into saucepan and bring to boil, slowly. Remove scum if necessary.
2. Simmer gently.
3. Rinse off barley well in sieve and add. Simmer for another 20 mins.
4. Add veg ½ an hour before serving and simmer.
5. Serve with fresh parsley on top.

Marinated and Stewed Rabbit

2-2.5 kg / 4-5 lb rabbit
½ cup wine vinegar
1 cup olive oil
1 chopped onion
1 sliced lemon
2 crumbed bay leaves
1 cup hot meat stock
Salt and pepper
2-3 anchovy fillets
3 Tbs softened butter
1 clove

Method
1. Clean rabbit and cut into serving pieces.
2. Put vinegar, half the oil, onion and lemon slices, clove and crushed bay leaves into a large bowl. Add rabbit, cover and leave for 24 hours in a cool place.
3. Remove lemon slices and stir rest of oil into marinade.
4. Put rabbit pieces into a pan with marinade and cook over low heat until browned.
5. Add stock, season lightly, cover pan and cook at low heat for one hour. Stir occasionally and add more stock if needed.
6. Chop anchovies and pound into butter. Add anchovy butter just before serving. Stir well.
7. Great with wild rice or new potatoes.

Apple Glazed Loin of Pork

Whole loin of pork 1.5 kg/3 lb
1/2 Tbs flour
1 tsp dry mustard
3 tsp salt
3/4 tsp pepper
1/8 tsp cloves

Glaze: 1 cup apple sauce or 2 stewed cooked apples
1 Tbs brown sugar
1/2 tsp cinnamon

Vegetables: Turnips, fennel and Lemon

Method:
1. Bone meat. Remove skin and score fat.
2. Mix mustard, flour, salt and pepper and rub well into inside and outside of meat.
3. Shape meat into a roll and tie with string.
4. Place on rack in roasting pan and roast at 160-180C/ 325-350F for 35 mins per 500g/1 lb and 30 mins extra.
5. Mix glaze ingredients and spread over meat halfway thru roasting period.
6. Cut skin into squares, place on rack with the meat and roast for 30 mins until crisp.

Wash and halve the fennel, sprinkle with lemon juice and season with sea salt and freshly ground black pepper and steam for 25 mins and serve with pork.

Boil chopped turnips for 15 mins. Drain and season with salt and pepper. Add a knob of butter and mash. Serve alongside fennel.

Mona's Spicy Meat balls

60g whole wheat bread crumbs
1 lb/ 500g minced free range beef
1 Tbs finely chopped onion
1/8 tsp all spice
¼ tsp pepper
45g/ 1 ½ oz butter
150 ml/ ¼ pint organic milk
1 beaten free range egg
¼ tsp mace (powdered)
1 tsp salt
Grated rind of one orange

Method:

1. Soak breadcrumbs in milk.
2. Mix crumbs with rest of ingredients aside from the butter. Shape into 12 balls.
3. Melt butter and fry balls until browned all over. Drain and set aside.

Mustard Sauce:

30g/ 1 oz flour
½ tsp salt
450 ml/ ¾ pint hot water
3 tsp mustard
1/8 tsp pepper

Method:

1. Mix flour, mustard, pepper and salt then add to pan in which you fried the meat balls.
2. Stir into left over butter with wooden spoon. Gradually add hot water and bring to boil.
3. Add meat balls, cover pan and simmer gently for ½ hour.

Roast Stuffed Pork Loin

1 loin of pork - 2.5 kg / 5 lb
1/2 cup cooked brown rice
1/2 cup chopped dried apricots
1 beef stock cube
1 cup water
1/4 cup pecan nuts
1/4 tsp mace
Tinned apricot halves

Apricot glaze: 3/4 c smooth apricot jam, 4 tsp lemon juice, 1/2 tsp ground cloves
 Combine and heat stirring until just boiling.

Method
1. Have the loin cut into chops joined loosely at bottom.
2. Combine rice, chopped apricots, stock cube and water in a saucepan.
Cook until rice is tender. Add more water if necessary.
3. Remove from heat and stir in chopped nuts and mace.
4. Insert a long skewer through top ends of chops to hold together. Place joint on a rack in a roasting pan.
5. Spoon rice stuffing between chops and cover tops loosely with foil. Roast at 160C / 325F for 2.5 hours.
6. Brush with glaze coating chops thinly.
7. Continue roasting, basting often with remaining glaze for another 1/2 hour. Pull out skewer and serve with tinned apricot halves.

4 fillets white fish ie turbot, hake.
6-8 rashers streaky bacon
2 onions sliced
3 Tbs butter
1/2 tsp mixed dried herbs
1 Tbs lovage chopped
Salt and pepper
2 Tbs flour
1 cup milk
3/4 cup grated cheddar
2 heaped Tbs whole wheat breadcrumbs
1 tomato skinned and sliced
Paprika

115g/ 4 oz kale
Olive oil
Garlic salt
Turmeric

Method:
1. Wipe fish off. Remove bacon rind and chop into 1 " lengths.
2. Sauté bacon and onions in 1 Tbs of the butter for 5 mins. Drain and place in oven proof dish.
3. Sprinkle with herbs (dried herbs and lovage) and lay fish on top - season well.
4. Melt remaining butter, stir in flour then remove from heat and gradually mix in milk. Return to heat and bring to boil stirring until sauce thickens. Add cheese to sauce, season and pour over fish.
5. Sprinkle with whole-wheat breadcrumbs and bake at 190c/375F for 30 mins.
6. After 15 mins layer sliced tomato on top and sprinkle with paprika.

Kale: Remove hard stems so you are left with the fleshy leaves. Place in a saucepan and drizzle with olive oil, then season well with salt and pepper. Sprinkle with garlic salt and turmeric and add 2-3 Tbs of water. Cover and cook for 10 mins, stirring occasionally. Remove lid and fry once water has evaporated for a more crispy result.

Serve fish with kale.

Lamb Cheeseburger

700 g / 24 oz minced lamb

2 Tbs bread crumbs
2 sprigs of Fresh Rosemary, leaves torn off
4 parsnips, sliced
4 carrots, sliced
4 chopped turnips

2 tsp curry powder

4-6 slices of tomato

Salt and pepper

Blue cheese or goat's cheese.

4 whole meal hamburger buns

Method:
1. Season the minced lamb with salt and ground black pepper and mix in breadcrumbs. Mix in rosemary and garlic well. Mold into four equal-sized patties, put on a plate cover in cling film and put them in the fridge for an hour.
2. Fry the burgers for 7-10 minutes on each side in canola oil until cooked. Set the burgers aside for a few minutes. Fry the slices of tomatoes in the same pan after seasoning with salt and pepper.
3. Boil the parsnips and carrots in a small amount of water with salt and curry powder. When soft: mash with butter.
4. Warm the burger buns

Serve the burgers on the buns topped with the fried tomato slices and some grated blue/goat's cheese. Place the mashed curried root veg at the side.

Lamb
600 gram Lamb shank
¾ cup Shiraz
½ cup organic plum vinegar
Fresh rosemary leaves
3 cloves of garlic

Method

1. Combine the rosemary, Shiraz, vinegar and garlic and marinate the lamb in it in a bag which you place in the fridge for 12 hours.
2. Remove lamb and place marinade in a pan to reduce until it become syrupy.
    Baste the lamb with the syrupy mixture and season with salt and pepper
3. Place it in the oven at 180C for about 20-25 mins or until cooked to your taste ie well done, rare.

Braised celery
2 heads celery
¼ onion thinly sliced
1 carrot thinly sliced
½ cup chicken stock
Salt and pepper
2 tsp butter
2 tsp flour

Method
1. Cut each stalk in half lengthways.
2. Place in pan of cold water, bring to boil and cook for 10 mins.
3. Drain, place in heavy bottomed saucepan with carrot, onion and chicken stock. Season, cover and cook slowly for 35-40 mins.

4. Mix butter and flour into a paste and stir into celery 5 mins before cooking time is up.

Mash
1 lb/500g Desire/red potatoes
3/4 cup coconut milk
Salt and ground black pepper
Smoked paprika
Dried Thyme

Method
1. Peel and then quarter potatoes
2. Steam potatoes for 25 mins
3. Mash with coconut milk, thyme and paprika.

Serve lamb with mash and braised celery.

Casserole of venison

¼ lb/ 115g bacon in one piece
2 lb/ 800g venison cut into small cubes
1 onion finely chopped
3 cloves garlic crushed
1 cup red wine
½ cup stock
2 bay leaves
2 cloves
¼ tsp each of rosemary, marjoram, thyme
Salt and pepper

Method
1. Cut rind from bacon and cut into small chunks. Sauté bacon gently for a few mins.
2. Transfer bacon to oven proof dish.
3. Coat venison pieces with flour and fry in bacon fat. Add onion garlic and continue frying for 3 more mins. Transfer to casserole dish with bacon.
4. Add stock and wine to pan and cook over high heat scrapping the crusty bits from bottom and sides.
5. Pour over venison.
6. Add bay leaves, cloves and herbs.
7. Season well and cook in a slow oven 150C/300F for 2-2.5 hours. Add stock as necessary.

Crab and Artichoke Casserole

1 bottle artichoke hearts
250-275g or 1/2- 3/4 lb fresh crab meat
1 small tin mushrooms or 7 oz fresh small mushrooms
2 Tbs butter
1 Tbs Worcestershire sauce
1/4 cup sherry
1 1/2 c white sauce *
1/4 c grated parmesan cheese

<u>White Sauce:</u> 2 Tbs butter, 2 Tbs Flour, 1 ½ cup milk.

Method:
1. Melt butter in a saucepan, removed from heat and stir in flour until a paste forms. Return to a low heat and stir in milk gradually. Stir until sauce thickens.
2. Drain artichoke hearts and arrange in a buttered corning dish.
3. Sprinkle crab meat over artichokes.
4. Drain mushrooms (or rinse if fresh) and saute in butter for 5 mins. Arrange over crab meat.
5. Add Worcestershire sauce and sherry to the white sauce, season and mix and pour over crab meat.
6. Top with grated cheese.
7. Bake at 180C for 20 mins.

Ingelegde Vis – Pickled Fish

500g/ 1lb fish
Canola Oil
1 tsp chillies
1 tsp turmeric
2 tsp curry
Chutney
Vinegar
1 large onion
1 tsp sugar
Salt
Orange or bay leaves

Method
1. Cut fish into 1 " slices and sprinkle with salt.
2. Fry fish in canola oil.
3. Slice onion and boil for a few mins in water.
4. Cover fish with vinegar. Add chillies, curry powder, turmeric and sugar and boil for a few mins. Cool.
5. Place fish into a deep earthenware jar in layers with the boiled onion.
6. Pour over curried sauce and cover. Within 2 days it will be ready for use.
7. Add orange or bay leaves on top of fish for added flavour.

Meatballs with Braised Cabbage and Mash

MeatBalls

1 lb/ 500g minced topside
1 large free range egg
1 cup oats
300 ml whole organic milk/soya milk
Ground ginger
All spice
Nutmeg
1 Tbs Worcestershire Sauce
1 Tbs wholemeal flour

Method
1. Soak the bread and oats in the milk and then mash.
2. Add the meat, beaten egg, flour and seasonings to the mash and mix well.
3. Shape into golf ball sized balls, roll in flour and fry until browned all over.

Gravy:
1. Sauté 1 large chopped onion in the oil left from the meat balls.
2. Add ½ cup beef stock and some ground black pepper and gravy seasoning if required.
3. Place meat balls into a casserole dish. Pour gravy over and simmer slowly for 30 mins.

Braised Cabbage

2-3 rashers bacon
1 large cabbage
Salt and pepper.
Nutmeg
3 cups stock
1 onion stuck with 2 cloves

1 large grated carrot
Bouquet Garni (parsley/thyme and bay leaf)

Method

1. Place bacon at bottom of pan and then divide cabbage into 8 pieces and place on top of bacon.
2. Sprinkle with salt, pepper and grated nutmeg.
3. Add onion, bouquet garni , carrot and stock.
4. Simmer for 1/2 hour.

Roast Duck Orange Sauce

1 duck
Salt and freshly ground black pepper
Lemon juice
1 small onion
1 small apple peeled and cored
Orange blossom Honey

Sauce
1 cup chicken stock
Juice of 2 oranges
1 cup cranberries
1 tsp orange rind
2 Tbs sherry
2 Tbs sugar
2 Tbs water

Optional: Chinese 5 Spice or Jamaican Jerk

Method

1. Season cavity of duck. Rub with lemon juice.
2. Cut apple and onion roughly and place inside duck
3. Cut criss-cross patterns in the skin and smear with honey, then season with salt and ground black pepper.
4. Place on rack of roasting pan and cook at 375F/ 190C for 20 mins per pound.
5. Baste occasionally with more honey.

Next:
1. Drain fat from roasting pan.
2. Add chicken stock to pan
3. Scrape excess from bottom and sides of pan and stir in.
4. Stir in orange juice, rind, cranberries and sherry.

5. In another saucepan caramelise the sugar with the water. (as in Crème Caramel recipe)
6. Add sugar to sauce and simmer gently until reduced to a syrupy consistency.

Carve duck and pour over sauce. If you feel adventurous add some Chinese 5 spice or Jamaican Jerk to the sauce for a real kick.

Roast Chicken with Baked Root Veg

1 whole free range or corn fed chicken
1 Tbs flour

2 peeled chopped parsnips
2 peeled chopped turnips
3 peeled chopped sweet potato or ½ pumpkin
1 Tbs oil
Vinegar
1 cup mayonnaise
1 cup peach chutney
salt and pepper

Stuffing
 2-3 slices Whole wheat bread sliced with crusts removed and soaked in water
 1 large onion grated
 ½ cup chopped fresh parsley
 1 beaten egg
 ¼ tsp dried thyme
 ¼ tsp dried sage
 Salt and ground black pepper

Method:

1. Rinse off chicken inside and out.
2. Mash soaked bread then mix with with onion, egg and herbs, until all the ingredients are well combined.
3. Place stuffing inside chicken.
4. Place chicken in an oven bag with 1 Tbs flour. It is best to put the flour in the bag first and shake it about.
5. Place on the rack in a roasting tin and cook for 20 mins per pound at 375F/ 190C.

Vegetables

1. Place peeled and roughly chopped vegetables into a roasting dish and toss in some oil.
2. Mix the mayonnaise and chutney together with some vinegar.
3. Coat the vegetable with the mixture.

Bake at 190C for 45mins to an hour. Remove halfway through and toss.

Slice and serve chicken with stuffing and root vegetables.

Rhubarbs with Meringue

3-4 sticks rhubarb

200g or 3/4 cup sugar

Meringue
2 egg whites
1 cup castor sugar
2 Tbs boiling water
1 tsp white vinegar
1/2 tsp vanilla essence
1 tsp baking powder

Method
1. Cut off ends of rhubarb. Cut into 1" pieces.
2. Place in a heavy based saucepan with the sugar and cover with water.
3. Simmer for 10 mins, stir occasionally to prevent sticking.
4. You will know rhubarb is done when it becomes mushy and the strings stick out.
5. Remove rhubarb and set aside.
6. You can make a syrup by boiling the remaining water while stirring, until the liquid becomes sticky and thick.

7. Combine all the meringue ingredients other than the baking powder.
8. Beat until stiff
9. Fold in the baking powder.
10. Place rhubarb in an oven proof dish and drizzle with the syrup.
11. Place spoonful's of meringue mixture on top of rhubarb and bake at 250F/120C for an hour.
12. Turn off oven and allow to dry out.

Serve with cream.

Rhubarb Trifle

1 packet raspberry or lemon-lime jello
1 sponge cake
1/2 cup sherry or Limoncello liquer
2 1/2c cold water
8 heaped Tbs milk powder
2 Tbs custard powder
Pinch salt
Whipping cream and chopped hazelnuts to decorate

Rhubarb: 200g or 3 stalks rhubarb cut into inch cubes
200g or 3/4 cup sugar
Water

Method
Note: You must begin this recipe either earlier on or the previous day to allow the jello to set.

1. Cut off ends of rhubarb.
2. Place in a heavy based saucepan with the sugar and cover with water.
3. Simmer for 10 mins, stir to prevent sticking occasionally.
4. You will know rhubarb is done when it becomes mushy and the strings stick out.
5. You can make syrup by boiling the remaining sugery water – keep an eye on it and stir often as it catches easily.

Mix up either the raspberry or lemon & lime jello as per instructions. Allow to cool then add rhubarb pieces. Refrigerate until jelly is firm.

Later on:

1. Make 600ml / 1 pint of custard by adding milk powder to the cold water with a pinch of salt and brining to the boil,

then adding the custard powder which you have made into a paste with some fresh milk.

2. Spread custard over the sponge cake which has been cut into portions over which sherry (if you use raspberry jello) or limoncello (if you use lemon and lime jello) was poured.
3. Allow to cool then place in fridge.

4. Remove jello (which has now set) from fridge and cut up into pieces.
5. Place pieces on top of cake and custard with some of the syrup from the rhubarb saucepan.

6. Put whipped cream and chopped hazelnuts on top. Refrigerate for 30 mins, then serve.

Banana Walnut Loaf

4 Tbs butter
1 cup castor sugar
1 large egg
1 cup mashed ripe banana
1/2 cup milk
2 1/2 cups flour
3 tsp baking power
1/4 tsp salt
1 cup walnuts chopped

Method

1. Cream butter and sugar until light and fluffy.
2. Add egg and beat until smooth.
3. Add bananas and milk and mix well.
4. Sift flour, baking powder and salt together and fold into banana mixture.
5. Fold in nuts.
6. Turn the mixture into a greased lined loaf tin 9x5 inches.
7. Bake for 1 hour at 350F/ 180C

Very Berry Ice Cream

500g / 1 lb berries (mix of raspberries, blueberries, cranberries) pureed and sieved
6 egg yolks
12 tsp sugar
600ml / 1 pint cream
Clear honey
Brandy
1 tsp cornflour

Method:

1. Beat egg yolks with sugar until thick
2. Beat in 6 Tbs berry pulp and the cream
3. Freeze for 6 hours
4. Make a sauce with remaining berries by heating and slightly thickening with corn flour. Stir while heating.
5. Add honey and a spoonful of brandy to sauce and serve hot with ice cream.

½ cup Granulated sugar
¼ cup unsalted butter
4 cups strawberries, raspberries, blueberries mixed.
2 tsp Lemon juice
Pinch salt

3 Tbs granulated sugar
4 Tbs water
3 large eggs
2 cups milk
Strawberry essence

Method
1. Add sugar and ¼ cup water to a saucepan and bring to the boil while stirring for 2 mins.
2. Add berries, lemon juice and salt.
3. Add butter and stir in until melted.
4. Remove from heat and spoon into the bottom of some molds.

Next:

1. Heat milk until hot, but not boiling. Pour milk over beaten eggs and sugar.
2. Add 2-3 drops strawberry essence and whisk.
3. Pour milk mixture into mold/s over fruit.
4. Stand mold/s in a larger basin filled with cold water and bake in center of oven at 275F/135C for 2 hours (If using individual molds cooking time is 1.5hours)

Creme caramel

3 Tbs granulated sugar
4 Tbs water
3 large eggs
2 cups milk
2-3 drops vanilla extract
Chopped Hazelnuts

Method

1. Put sugar and half the water into a small heavy saucepan over low heat.
2. Cook stirring until sugar dissolves
3. Raise heat and boil until liquid turns golden brown, watch carefully as it can burn.
4. Remove from heat and add remaining water; the caramel will boil fast and furiously and become a sticky ball.
5. Return to heat and stir until it becomes liquid again.
6. Grease a mould and pour caramel in.
7. Pop the hazelnuts into the mould on top of caramel.
8. Heat milk until hot, but not boiling. Pour milk over beaten eggs and sugar. Mix. Sprinkle in vanilla.
9. Pour milk mixture into moulds.
10. Stand mould in a larger basin filled with cold water and bake in centre of oven at 275F/ 135C for 2 hours (If using individual moulds cooking time is 1.5 hours)

Bibliography

Denmark Author. (2010, January 31). *Food and Drink.* Retrieved from
    Denmark: http://denmark.dk/en/lifestyle/food-drink/

Dr. Thomas Meinert Larsen, e. a. (2012, November 5-7). *University of
    Copenhagen.* Retrieved from Health Benefits of the New Nordic
    Diet:
    http://nynordiskmad.org/fileadmin/webmasterfiles/Arkiv/fil
    er/121106_Thomas%20Meinert%20Larsen_NNM%20konfere
    nce_Oslo.pdf

Hansen, J. L. (2012, March 3). *Focus Denmark.* Retrieved from Demark:
    http://denmark.dk/en/lifestyle/food-drink/redzepis-recipe/

Medianet author. (June, 2013 1). *Nordic Diet.* Retrieved from Media
    Net:
    http://www.medindia.net/patients/lifestyleandwellness/nord
    ic-diet.htm

MedIndia. (2015, January 17). *Nordic Diet.* Retrieved from
    MedIndia.net:
    http://www.medindia.net/patients/lifestyleandwellness/nord
    ic-diet.htm#ixzz3P2wo95nh

Siddique, A. (2013, May 30). *Nordic Diet Plan, like Mediterranean,
    Lowers Cholestrol and Inflammation.* Retrieved from Medical
    Daily: http://www.medicaldaily.com/nordic-diet-plan-
    mediterranean-lowers-cholesterol-and-inflammation-246380

Made in the USA
San Bernardino, CA
19 May 2016